TABLE OF CONTENT.

8. **Conclusion**
- Recap of Vegetarian Diet Benefits and Drawbacks
- Importance of a Balanced Diet
- Final Thoughts on Vegetarianism.

Prologue TO

The Veggie BOOK

(A total aide for veggie lover feast plan).

Vegan diets might be related with a few medical advantages and further developed diet quality. Nonetheless, legitimate arranging is vital to forestall dietary inadequacies and adverse consequences on wellbeing.

The veggie lover diet has acquired far reaching ubiquity as of late.

A few examinations gauge that veggie lovers represent around 6% and 5% of the populace in North America and Europe, separately, while around 19% of the populace in Asia is vegan.

Aside from the moral and ecological purposes behind cutting meat from your eating routine, a very much arranged vegan diet may likewise decrease your gamble of ongoing illness, support weight reduction, and work on the nature of your eating regimen.

This article gives a novice's manual for the veggie lover diet, including an example feast plan for multi week.

What is a veggie lover diet?

The vegan diet includes keeping away from eating meat, fish, and poultry.

Individuals frequently take on a vegan diet for strict or individual reasons, as well as moral issues, like basic entitlements.

Others choose to become veggie lover for ecological reasons, as domesticated animals creation increments ozone harming substance emanations, adds to environmental change, and requires a lot of water, energy, and normal assets.

There are a few types of vegetarianism, every one of which varies in their limitations.

The most well-known types include:

- Lacto-ovo-vegan diet: kills meat, fish, and poultry however permits eggs and dairy items

- Lacto-vegan diet: kills meat, fish, poultry, and eggs however permits.

- Ovo-vegan diet: kills meat, fish, poultry, and dairy items however permits eggs.

- Pescatarian diet: kills meat and poultry however permits fish and once in a while eggs and dairy items

- Veggie lover diet: dispenses with meat, fish, poultry, eggs, and dairy items, as well as other creature determined items, like honey.

- Flexitarian diet: a for the most part vegan diet that consolidates infrequent meat, fish, or poultry

A great many people who follow a vegan diet don't eat meat, fish or poultry. Different varieties include the consideration or avoidance of eggs, dairy, and other creature items.

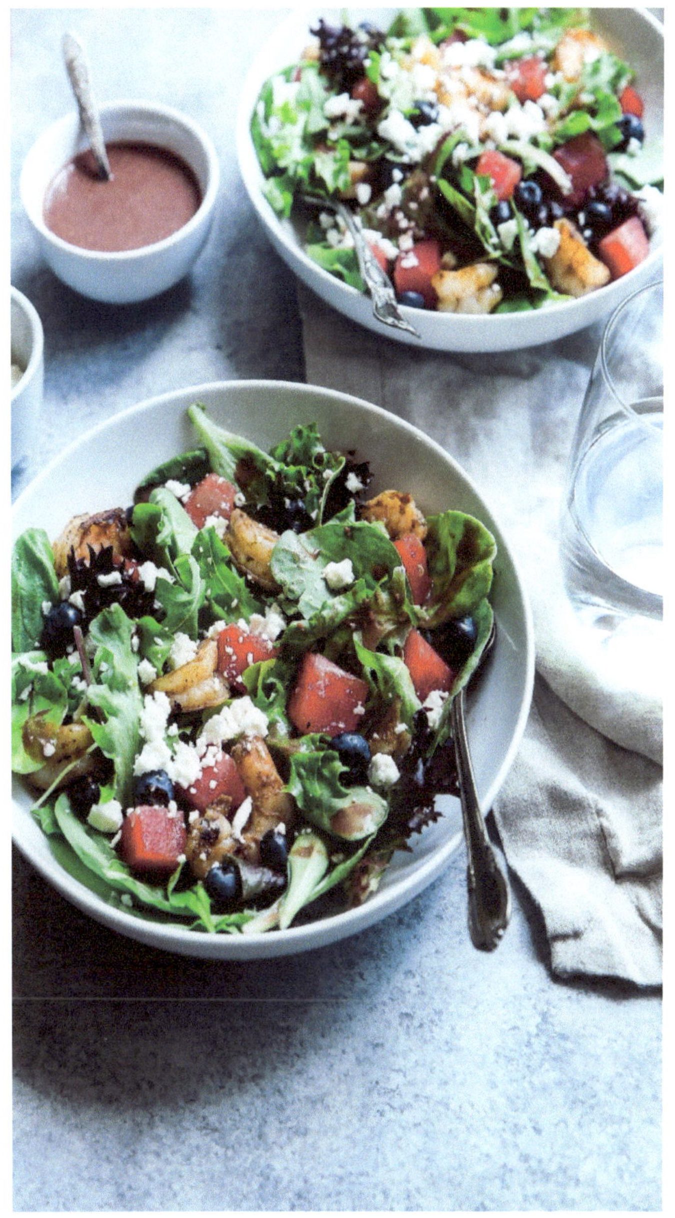

HEALTH BENEFITS.

Here are few health benefits of a vegan or veggie meals:

Medical advantages;

Veggie lover slims down are related with various medical advantages.

As a matter of fact, concentrates on show that vegans will generally have preferable eating routine quality over meat-eaters and a higher admission of significant supplements like fiber L-ascorbic acid, vitamin E, and magnesium A veggie lover diet might give a few other wellbeing supports too.

Upgrades weight reduction;

Changing to a vegan diet can be a compelling technique in the event that you're hoping to free weight.

By and large, experienced 4.5 more pounds (2 kilograms) of weight reduction north of 18 weeks than non-veggie lovers.

Essentially, a 6-month concentrate on in 74 individuals with type 2 diabetes exhibited that vegan eats less were almost two times as successful at decreasing body weight as low-calorie diet. Besides, a recent report in almost 61,000 grown-ups showed that veggie lovers will generally have a lower weight file (BMI) than omnivores — BMI being an estimation of muscle versus fat in light of level and weight. Notwithstanding, more examination is expected to comprehend which explicit parts of the veggie lover diet or way of life might be answerable for this affiliation.

Diminishes disease risk;

Some exploration proposes that a veggie lover diet might be connected to a lower chance of disease including those of the bosom, colon, and rectum. Nonetheless, ebb and flow research is restricted to observational examinations, which can't demonstrate a circumstances and logical results relationship. Remember that a few examinations have turned up conflicting discoveries. Hence, more exploration is expected to comprehend what vegetarianism might mean for disease risk.

Balances out glucose;

A few examinations demonstrate that vegan diets might assist with keeping up with solid glucose levels.

For example, one 2014 survey of six examinations connected vegetarianism to further developed glucose control in individuals with type 2 diabetes Vegan diets may likewise forestall diabetes by balancing out glucose level in the long haul.

As per one concentrate in 2,918 individuals, changing from a non-veggie lover to a vegan diet was related with a 53% diminished hazard of diabetes over a normal of 5 years.

Advances heart wellbeing

Veggie lover eats less carbs diminish a few coronary illness risk variables to assist with keeping your heart sound areas of strength for and.

One ongoing survey found that veggie lover diets could prompt a little decrease in all out cholesterol and LDL (terrible) cholesterol levels, the two of which are risk factors for coronary illness.

Nonetheless, a similar survey likewise found that veggie lover slims down prompted an expansion in fatty oils and a decrease in HDL (great) cholesterol levels contrasted with other dietary mediations

Likewise, one more concentrate in 118 individuals found that a low-calorie vegan diet was more successful at lessening LDL (terrible) cholesterol than a Mediterranean eating routine. Then again, the Mediterranean eating regimen prompted a more prominent decrease in fatty substance levels. Other examination shows that vegetarianism might be related with lower circulatory strain levels. Hypertension is another key gamble factor for coronary illness

In any case, research has turned up blended results. In this manner, more examinations are expected to decide if veggie lover eats less really decrease the gamble of creating or passing on from coronary illness.

Taking everything into account;

Besides the fact that veggie lovers will generally have a higher admission of a few key supplements, yet vegetarianism has been related with weight reduction, diminished disease risk, further developed glucose, and better heart wellbeing. Be that as it may, more examination is required.

Expected drawbacks;
A balanced vegan diet can be sound and nutritious.

Be that as it may, it might likewise build your gamble of specific wholesome lacks.

Meat, poultry and fish supply a lot of protein and omega-3 unsaturated fats, as well as micronutrients prefer zinc, selenium, iron, and vitamin B12.

Other creature items like dairy and eggs additionally contain a lot of calcium, vitamin D, and B nutrients.

While cutting meat or other creature items from your eating regimen, it's vital to guarantee you're getting these fundamental supplements from different sources.

Concentrates on show that veggie lovers are at a higher gamble of protein, calcium, iron, iodine, and vitamin B12 inadequacies.

A lack of dietary in these key micronutrients can prompt side effects like weariness, shortcoming, iron deficiency, bone misfortune, and thyroid, including different organic products, vegetables, entire grains, protein sources, and sustained food varieties is a simple method for guaranteeing you're getting fitting sustenance.

Multivitamins and enhancements are one more choice to rapidly knock up your admission and make up for possible lacks.

All in all;

Removing meat and creature-based items can build your gamble of dietary inadequacies. An even eating routine — conceivably close by supplements — can assist with forestalling lacks.

Food varieties TO EAT

A veggie lover diet ought to incorporate a different blend of organic products, vegetables, grains, sound fats, and proteins.

To supplant the protein given by meat in your eating routine, incorporate an assortment of protein-rich plant food varieties like entire grains, vegetables, tempeh, tofu, and seitan.

On the off chance that you follow a lacto-ovo-vegan diet, eggs and dairy can likewise support your protein consumption.

Eating supplement thick entire food sources like organic products, vegetables, and entire grains will supply a scope of significant nutrients and minerals to fill in any healthful holes in your eating routine.

A couple of quality food sources to eat on a vegan diet are:

•	Natural products: apples, bananas, berries, oranges, melons, pears, peaches

•	Vegetables: salad greens, asparagus, broccoli, tomatoes, carrots

•	Grains: quinoa, grain, buckwheat, rice, oats

•	Vegetables: lentils, beans, peas, chickpeas

•	Nuts: almonds, pecans, cashews, chestnuts

•	Seeds: flaxseed, chia, and hemp seeds

•	Solid fats: olive oil, avocados

•	Proteins: tempeh, tofu, seitan, natto, nourishing yeast, spirulina, eggs, dairy items

All in all;

A solid vegan diet incorporates different nutritious food varieties like organic products, vegetables, grains, sound fats, and plant-based proteins.

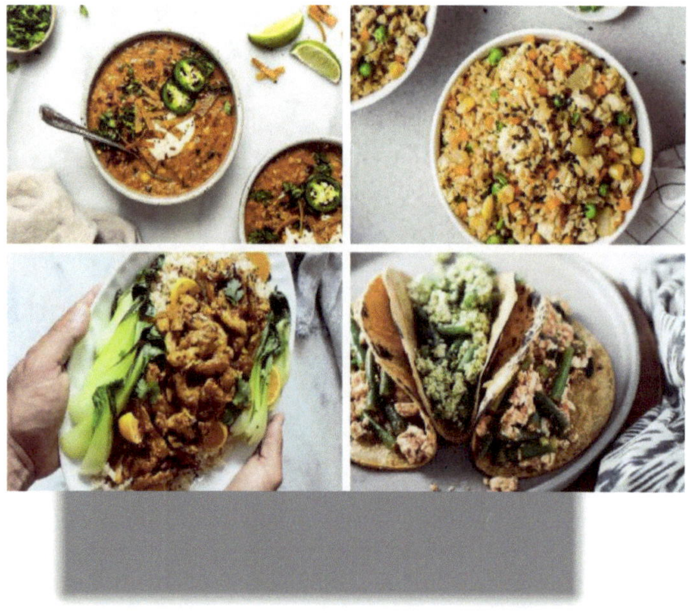

Food sources TO Stay away from:

There are numerous varieties of vegetarianism, each with various limitations.

Lacto-ovo vegetarianism, the most widely recognized kind of vegan diet, includes taking out all meat, poultry, and fish.

Different sorts of vegans may likewise stay away from food varieties like eggs and dairy.

A veggie lover diet is the most prohibitive type of vegetarianism since it bars meat, poultry, fish, eggs, dairy, and some other creature items.

Contingent upon your requirements and inclinations, you might need to keep away from the accompanying food varieties on a vegan diet:

- Meat: hamburger, veal, and pork

- Poultry: chicken and turkey

- Fish and shellfish: This limitation doesn't have any significant bearing to pescatarians.

- Meat-based fixings: gelatin, fat, carmine, isinglass, oleic corrosive, and suet

- Eggs: This limitation applies to veggie lovers and lacto-vegans.

- Dairy items: This limitation on milk, yogurt, and cheddar applies to veggie lovers and ovo-vegans.

- Other creature items: Vegetarians might decide to keep away from honey, beeswax, and dust.

All in all;

Most vegans stay away from meat, poultry, and fish. Certain varieties of vegetarianism may likewise confine eggs, dairy, and other creature items.

Test dinner plan

To assist with kicking you off, here's a **1-week test dinner plan for a lacto-ovo-vegan diet.**

Monday

•	Breakfast: cereal with natural product, nut spread, flaxseed, and a glass of soy milk

•	Lunch: barbecued veggie and hummus wrap on an entire grain tortilla with lentil salad

•	Supper: tofu banh mi sandwich with cured slaw.

Tuesday

- Breakfast: fried eggs with tomatoes, garlic, and mushrooms

- Lunch: zucchini boats loaded down with flavored lentils, veggies, and feta with a side of tomato soup

- Supper: chickpea curry with basmati rice.

Wednesday

- Breakfast: Greek yogurt with chia seeds and berries

- Lunch: faro salad with tomatoes, cucumber, and feta with flavored lentil soup

- Supper: eggplant parmesan and barbecued seitan with a side serving of mixed greens

Thursday

- Breakfast: tofu scramble with sautéed peppers, onions, and spinach

- Lunch: burrito bowl with earthy colored rice, beans, avocado, salsa, and veggies

- Supper: vegetable paella with heated tempeh a side plate of mixed greens

Friday

- Breakfast: entire wheat toast finished off with avocado, chickpeas, and nourishing yeast

- Lunch: marinated tofu pita pocket with Greek serving of mixed greens

- Supper: quinoa-dark bean meatballs with zucchini noodles

Saturday

- Breakfast: smoothie of kale, berries, bananas, nut margarine, almond milk, and a scoop of plant-based protein powder

- Lunch: dark bean veggie burger on an entire grain bun with avocado serving of mixed greens

- Supper: entire grain flatbread with flavored lentils, barbecued garden vegetables, and pesto

Sunday

- Breakfast: kale and yam hash

- Lunch: ringer peppers loaded down with tempeh with zucchini wastes

- Supper: dark bean tacos with cauliflower rice

All in all;

above is an example menu of what multi week on a lacto-ovo-vegan diet might seem to be. This plan can be adapted to different styles of vegetarianism too.

MEATLESS MONDAY 6 WEEK MEAL PLAN

	BREAKFAST	LUNCH	SNACK	DINNER
Week 1	Overnight Oats	Black Bean Burrito	Everything Chickpeas	Alfredo Pasta
Week 2	Breakfast Sweet Potato	BBQ Veggie Bowl	Black Bean Dip	Crunchy Lentil Tacos
Week 3	Tofu Scramble	Kidney Bean Curry	Spicy Cashew 'Cheese' Dip	Eggplant Meatballs
Week 4	Peanut Butter & Banana Toast	'Chick'n' Caesar Wrap	Hummus & Veggie Sticks	Burrito Bowl
Week 5	Fruit & Veggie Protein Smoothie	Kale & Grain Salad	PB&J Banana Roll-Ups	Tuscan Veggie Pasta
Week 6	Avocado Toast with 'Sausage' Patty	Protein-Packed Chili Nachos	Popcorn with Nutritional Yeast	Veggie Zoodle Pad Thai

Conclusion/End

Most vegans keep away from meat, poultry, and fish; however, some likewise limit eggs, dairy, and other creature items.

A fair vegan diet with nutritious food varieties like produce, grains, sound fats, and plant-based protein might offer a few advantages, however it might expand your gamble of healthful lacks if misguided.

Make certain to consider a couple of key supplements and balance your eating routine with different solid entire food varieties. Like that, you'll partake in the advantages of vegetarianism while limiting the secondary effects.

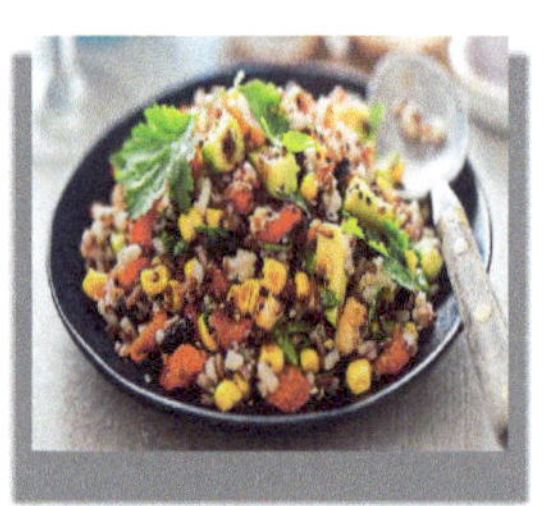
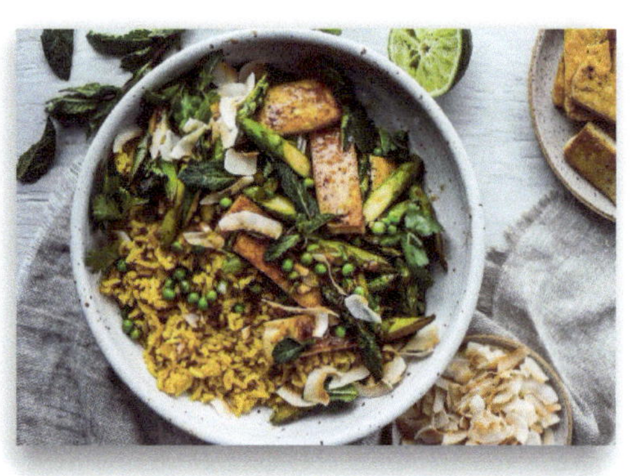
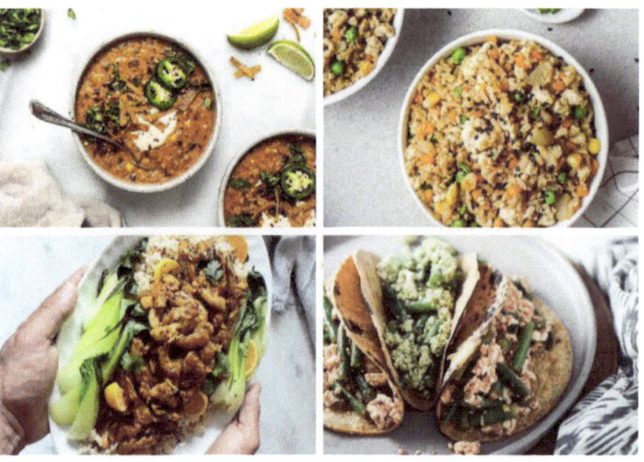